€8

HOMOEOPATHIC TREATMENT FOR E.N.T. DISEASES

by

Dr. S.G. Palsule, D.M.S.

B. Jain Publishers (P) Ltd.

New Delhi

Reprint edition : 2000

Price: Rs. 15.00

Published by :
Kuldeep Jain
For
B. Jain Publishers (P.) Ltd.
1921, Street No. 10, Chuna Mandi,
Paharganj, New Delhi 110 055 (INDIA)
Phones: 3670430; 3670572; 7536418
FAX 011-3610471 & 7536420
Email: bjain@vsnl.com

Printed in India by:
Unisons Techno Financial Consultants (P) Ltd.
522, FIE, Patpar Ganj, Delhi - 110 092

ISBN : 81-7021-802-0
BOOK CODE: BS-2407

PREFACE

(1st Edition)

I have great pleasure in introducing a concise book on the diseases of the Ear, Nose and Throat with their homoeopathic treatment. I felt it very necessary to have such a book on these specialised subjects where many of the homoeopathic practitioners face difficulties in treating the kind of cases described in this booklet.

This book is also useful to allopathic and ayurvedic physicians who need correct guidance & scientific approach to these subjects.

The E. N. T. surgeon also can refer to this booklet and decide whether the case is surgical or medical in nature, prior to operation.

The essential therapeutic use of the medicines is given under different chapters. The characteristic symptoms of each medicine are described, though for the full recognition of symptoms the help of the standard Materia

Medica is highly essential. The additional description of the medicines will simply increase the size and price of the book.

(3rd Edition)

It is gratifying to note that this book on E.N.T. runs into its third edition. A new chapter on sinusitis and its homoeopathic treatment is added to the third edition. It was left unnoticed in the earlier editions due to my preoccupations and, therefore, has been taken after the throat diseases.

My other books like Asthma and Blood Pressure, Lights on Homoeopathic Potency, Dentistry & Homoeopathy in English and other Marathi books are also selling well, which shows the wider interest of the medical practitioners and general readers on the subject.

Dr. S. G. Palsule

SOME SUGGESTIONS

I would like to throw some light on using potencies while prescribing the homoeopathic medicines.

Practically, there is no hard and fast rule about using different potencies. Still the masters in this line like Dr. Hahnemann, Dr. Boericke, Dr. Kent and many other celebrated homoeopaths have shown us the correct path regarding selection of the potency. Dr. Hahnemann has done his provings mostly with 30 potency. Dr. Close opines that higher the susceptibility, higher the potency. Thus small children who are highly susceptible, that is to say quick to react to the medicinal action, require higher potencies. In this manner, 200 and 1000 potencies can be used wherever necessary. If the sensations of the patient have become numb due to different causes, lower potencies should be given such as 3 or 6 or even mother tincture.

For repetition of doses, again the susceptibility of the patient is the guide. In acute cases and severe cases it is always better to judge the patient's general condition and then confirm the potency. In chronic cases, especially with skin diseases, higher potencies should be selected and given after four, eight, 15 days or a month's duration. Personally 1 have experienced that 30 & 200 potencies are adequate to cover most of the common ailments. In organic diseases lower potencies and in functional disorders higher potencies can generally be used. Medicines to be given in alteration also have a sure place in homoeopathy. This method is only followed when a medicine partially covers the totality of symptoms of a given case and the second one to be chosen covers the rest of the symptoms and at the same time does not antidote the effects of the former one.

Contents

EAR DISEASES

OTITIS MEDIA

In diseases of the ear, we often observe the condition of discharges from the ear. The inflammation of the middle year is know as 'Otitis Media', which is primarily the outcome of a tube-tympanic catarrh.

Acute causes

Various conditions of the nose and nasopharynx by extension of the common cold or infection.

In children, adenoid growth, enlarged and

septic tonsils are frequently the primary causes of acute middle ear involvement.

Measles, typhoid fever, influenza and pneumonia are also the contributory causes for acute otitis media.

Pyorrhoea, injury or accident also help to cause the discharge.

Syphilis, tuberculosis, anaemia, kidney disease must be sought for as the possible causes for the continuance of chronic otitis media.

A bloody discharge may be due to *Streptococcus haemolyticus* infection.

If the acute condition of the ear discharge is not properly treated, it passes into, a chronic condition.

Treatment

Ferrum phos

Suits well when there is an inflammation, congestion and pain. The discharge is mucopurulent in nature. It is useful in the first stage, of all acute specific fevers with symptoms of otitis media.

Capsicum

Is indicated when there is a rupture of the ear drum, and great soreness of the mastoid portion. The ears are hot and the pain goes to the throat. The drum is perforated and the discharge is yellow, purulent.

Mercurius vivus

Is very useful when there is swelling of parotid glands. It suits well to scrofulous and syphilitic ear conditions. Offensive breathe, enlarged tonsils and night aggravation are its other characteristics. It should be used in 6, 10 or 200 potencies.

Hepar sulph

Ear trouble with enlarged tonsils. Cold and sore throat. Cures boils in the ear and useful in mastoiditis. 200 and 1000 potencies work well.

Silicea

Caries or necrosis of the bones with a thin, ichorous offensive discharge containing little pieces of bone. Perforated ear drum. Persistent chronic discharges from the ear. Use 200 and 1000 potencies in chronic cases and 6 or 30 in acute disease.

OTALGIA

Otalgia or pain in the ear occurs in all acute inflammatory conditions of the ear with acute exacerbation of chronic suppurative conditions. Pain due to reflex cause is also a factor. Carious teeth, ulceration of the pharynx, tonsils or larynx may cause pain in the ear. The pain of acute otitis externa is aggravated by motions of the jaw, as in chewing. Pain is usually constant. In such cases, the patient is very sensitive to examination due to pain. The pain of a middle ear condition is worse by swallowing, belching, talking or any act which causes movement of the tissues of the eustachian tube. It lacks the aggravation of the pain of external otitis. Patient is not sensitive to examination. The pain of a mastoid affection is deep and boring in the region of the mastoid.

Treatment

Aconite

When the external ear is inflamed, red and swollen with pain. Acute symptoms.

Belladonna

The pains come and go suddenly. Pain in the ear with headache and red face, throbbing of carotids etc. It is useful in both otitis interna and externa. Parotid glands are swollen with otitis media. Blood boil in the ear and throbbing pain call for this remedy.

Chamomilla

Is useful when the pains are violent, worse, from warmth. Aggravation at night and from slightest cold. The child is very restless, crying and remains calm when carried by the mother. Ear pain during dentition.

Arnica

Suits well when the pain is in the cartilages of the ear. Pain is as if bruised or due to injury.

Mullein Oil

The use of this oil while going to bed or during pain by instillation of the drops has a soothing effect. Two or three drops are to be instilled in the affected ear.

Apis

Is useful in puffy swelling and stinging pains with shining redness of the ear.

Use 6, 30, potency for acute cases and 200 or 1000 for chronic cases.

MASTOIDITIS

Causes

- Acute and Chronic Otitis Media.

- Direct trauma (injury) may cause primary mastoiditis.

Infection causes pus, stagnation and necrosis of bone.

The accumulation of debris within the mastoid, causes erosion and consequently an abscess is formed in the area. Extradural abscess, meningitis or sinus thrombosis may occur as complications. In haemorrhagic mastoiditis, thrombosis in the smaller vascular channels takes place. It is due to *Streptococcus haemolyticus*.

Symptoms

In acute mastoiditis, pain and tenderness is observed. It is usually constant, dull and boring in character. This symptom is more prominent in children than in adults. The intensity depends upon the virulency of the infection. When the mastoid capsule ruptures, the pain stops. On account of this cessation of pain, the physician is apt to think of improvement. Sleeplessness is a symptom, in many patients, of acute mastoiditis. The sleeplessness has no direct connection with the pain. The symptoms vary according to the stage and the portion occupied in mastoiditis. Oedema over the mastoid occurs when the outer plate is involved. Comparison with the other mastoid is an aid in diagnosis. After the rupture takes place, prominence of the auricle is seen. It is due to pus and oedematous tissue. In chronic mastoiditis, no special subjective symptoms are present and hence it, is necessary to examine the patient thoroughly well.

Symptoms of chronic mastoiditis

Headache is referred to the parietal and frontal regions of the affected side. Photophobia is noted in the beginning of meningeal condition. Mental excitement and restlessness with a desire to get out of bed etc. will be seen.

Examination of blood for white cell counts and differential counts is helpful.

General Treatment

Wide open drainage and checking of otitis media is very important. If the discharge is purulent, mastoid operation is called for. X-Ray examination helps in confirmation.

Treatment

Capsicum

Is useful in otitis media with rupture of the drum. There is great soreness of the mastoid portion of the temporal bone. It cures chronic suppuration. The ears are hot and pain shifts to the throat. It cures yellow, purulent discharge.

Aurum met

For fetid discharge, boring, pain in the mastoid, caries and perforated drum. Suits well in syphilitic constitutions.

Calcarea carb

Is useful in chronic ear trouble, especially in

scrofulous children. Itching in the ears with purulent discharge.

Other Medicines

Hepar sulph. and Mercurius v. (see the symptoms under otitis media) are also useful medicines. Fluoric acid and Asafoetida should be considered while treating the cases of mastoiditis.

TINITUS

This condition is characterised by head noises which are basically associated with the inner ear. The character of the sound may be buzzing, roaring, hammering, hissing etc.. These symptoms are felt by the patient. Drugs like quinine, salicylates cause noises in the ear. High blood pressure, rheumatic ailments, otitis media, labyrinthitis, osteosclerosis are the causative factors of tinitus.

Treatment

Salicylic acid

Simple deafness with tinitus. Roaring in the ears and ringing sounds. Vertigo. Potency 6 or 30

Causticum

Roaring in the ears, buzzing sound especially when there is eustachian catarrh. Words and steps re-echo. Potency 200.

Chininum sulph.

When there is a malarial history with violent ringing and roaring. It suits well in gouty or rheumatic subjects. Potency 6 and 30.

Glonoin

Tinitus with high blood premure. Potency 200.

Lachesis

Tinitus while going to bed and the patient is worse after sleep. Potency 30 or 200.

MYRINGITIS

Myringitis means the inflammation of the tympanic membrane. This membrane is composed of three layers Outer (dermal), Central (fibrous) and Inner (mucous layer). These tissues are liable to inflammation. The ear drum is situated between the middle ear cavity and the external canal. The average case of myringitis is secondary to the inflammatory conditions of either the external or middle ear. It is rarely a primary condition. The medicines for meningitis are:-

Aconite; Belladonna, Hepar sulph, Sulphur etc.

Symptoms of these common medicines can be seen in the standard homoeopathic materia medica and under some chapters in this booklet.

NOSE DISEASES

EPISTAXIS

Epistaxis means bleeding from the nose. It is due to local and general causes.

Causes

Congestion of the mucous membrane such as that which accompanies adenoids, polypi, acute rhinitis, worms in the nose, mechanical injuries (directly or indirectly), foreign body in the nose etc. Malignant disease, syphilis, tuberculosis and ulcerations are also factors. When the blood is not much in quantity, it may pass backward into the throat and is swallowed or expectorated or coughed up. This may lead to an erroneous diagnosis of haemoptysis or hematemesis. In chronic nephritis or high blood pressure, there is nose-bleed. It frequently occurs in valvular disease of the heart, emphysema, chronic bronchitis, liver cirrhosis, extremes of temperature and thoracic tumors etc. Violent exercise, menstrual period, mountaineering also cause nose bleed. Haemophilia, scurvy, leukemia, anaemia, thrombocytopenia are conditions of altered blood states in which epistaxis takes place. Specific fever such as typhoid, rheumatism, haemorrhagic forms of exanthema and whooping cough cause nose bleed.

Treatment

Arnica

Is useful in traumatic epistaxis. Potency 30, 200.

Ammonium carb

Blood appears from the nose on blowing or washing it. There is congestive cold. After eating there is nose bleed. Ozena, blows bloody mucus from nose, Potency 6 or 200.

Ambrosia

Blood from the nose due to cold, rhinitis and whooping cough. Also useful in bronchitis with nose bleed. Potency 3 or 6.

Ferrum phos

Bright red blood flow from the nose with congestion, headache and cold. Bleeding from the nose due to sunstroke, anaemia, high blood pressure etc. Potency 6, 30 or 200.

Ipecacuanha

Suits well in epistaxis especially when its characteristic symptom of nausea and vomiting is present. Blood is bright red and comes from any part of the body. Epistaxis due to bronchitis, emphysema, tuberculosis and abdominal diseases call for its use. Potency 30 or 200.

Millefolium

Bright red blood from mechanical injuries. Potency 6 or 30.

Other Medicines

Hamamelis, China, Erigeron and Melilotus are also useful medicines in cases of epistaxis. Arsenic can be given in malignant disease. Cina works well in wormy children.

POLYPI

Polypi are the most frequent new growths in the nose. Three known kinds of polypi are (1) Mucous (2) Nasopharyngeal and (3) Malignant (cancerous). Mucous polypi are mostly oedematous mucosa. There is often an allergic constitution Polypi may be found in both the nostrils. The size and extent of polypi may vary from a few small beads along the under surface of the middle turbinate bone to enormous masses completely filling both nostrils. In asthma and frequent cases of coryza, polypi are pedunculated, pale, grey, glistening bodies. Septic infection is one of the causes for polypi.

Naso-pharyngeal polypi are rarely seen. It is the fibroma of the naso-pharynx. It may expand the bones of the face causing deformity known as "frog face".

The main symptoms are nasal obstruction, discharge and bleeding from the nose.

Malignant polypi are rare. They also cause "frog-face". They are often accompanied by glands in the neck, pain, bleeding and offensive discharge.

Fibroma and cancerous growths require surgical treatment.

Treatment

Sanguinaria nitrate

Is useful in acute and chronic catarrh with polypus in the nose. It cures acute pharyngitis. Nose feels obstructed. There is profuse, watery mucus with burning pain. Enlarged turbinates at the beginning of the hypertrophic process. Small crusts in the nose which bleed when removed. Dry and burning nostrils. Sneezing, Potency 3, 6 or 200.

Lemna minor

Cures nasal polypi with swollen turbinates. It is a very useful medicine in atrophic rhinitis. It removes oedematous condition of the polypi thereby relieving the obstruction. Potency 3.

Cadmium sulph

It is very useful in ozena. Polypus, caries of the nasal bones, boils on the nose, ulcerated nostrils etc. are cured. Potency 6 or 30.

Other medicines

Sabadilla, Teucrium, Calcarea carb and Formica should be given in cases of polypus if symptoms call for the use of these remedies.

RHINITIS

Rhinitis means inflammation of the nasal mucous membrane. It is set up by irritation of any kind such as dust vapour or foreign body like pea or marble inserted in the nose. The commonest cause is a "Cold." In acute coryza or "Cold in the head" there is a profuse mucopurulent discharge attended by sneezing, running from the eyes and feverishness with frontal headache. It is also produced by droplet infection. Rhinitis is also caused by adenoids, septic tonsils, sinus troubles and cold or damp weather.

Chronic rhinitis is a chronic inflammatory condition of the mucous membrane of the nose attended by increased secretion and usually thickening of the area. Simple, hypertrophic and atrophic forms are known to exist. It presents the same symptoms of acute form but in a greater degree. Even in milder form, patient suffers from headache and mental depression. It is frequently associated with adenoids.

Chronic maxillary sinusitis is the commonest form of sinusitis. Chronic sinusitis is due to an extension of infection from the cavities of the nose. Influenza is responsible for many cases. It may arise after specific fevers, injury or operation of the nose. "Cold in. the head" is the most frequent cause of chronic sinusitis. The offensive discharge from the nose is called ozena or atrophic rhinitis. Syphilis and cancer are the two diseases which cause atrophic rhinitis. Faceache or neuralgia of the face may result from sinusitis.

Treatment

Aconite

Is useful in acute and sudden cold. Cold caused by exposure to dry cold weather, checked perspiration or influenza. There is pain at the root of nose. Rhinitis with much sneezing. Mucous membrane dry, nose stopped up. Dry or slight watery coryza.. Potency 200 and 1000.

Ammonium carb

Discharge of sharp burning water. Stoppage of nose at night with long continued coryza. Difficulty in breathing, sneezing. Nose bleed after washing, the face & after eating. Ozena, tip of the nose congested. For patients using smelling bottles (nasal sprays). Potency 6 or 200.

Arsenic

Thin, watery, excoriating discharge. Sneezing without relief. Nightly aggravation. Hay fever, worse in open air. Lupus of the nose. Potency 200.

Sabadilla

Coryza with severe frontal pains, redness of the eyes with watering (lachrymation). Copious, watery nasal discharge. sneezing chronic complaints of cold. Potency 6 or 200.

Solidago vera

Is useful for repeated colds or tuberculosis. Feeling of weakness, chilliness alternating with heat, nasopharyngeal cold. Chest feels oppressed. Hay fever. Potency 3 or 6.

ATROPHIC RHINITIS

Arsenic, Iodide, Hepar sulph, Hippzaenia, Kali bichromicum, Pulsatilla and Sepia should be given according to symptoms.

HYPERTROPHIC RHINITIS

In hypertrophic rhinitis, the most prominent symptom is difficult nasal breathing due to hypertrophic (thickened) condition of the tissues and due to the thick tenacious secretion. The closing of the nostril is most noticeable when lying down and causes "mouth breathing". The sense of smell is diminished or wholly lost and the sense of taste is frequently impaired. Periodical frontal headache is a marked symptom which is neuralgic in character. Chronic hypertrophic rhinitis also cause tinnitus and deafness to some extent.

Arum triphyllum Aralia, Kali bichromicum, Aurum met, Pulsatilla, Kali sulph are useful medicines.

SINUSITIS

Sinus trouble or Sinusitis is observed frequently. People who live in temperate or cold climates, mostly suffer from this trouble. Seasonal and even daily changes of weather often have an adverse effect upon the sinus trouble.

The nasal sinuses are part of the respiratory system. These are cavities in the face and skull bones, where inspired air is slightly warmed before proceeding in the lungs. The cavities are linked with mucous membranes, like the canals of the nostrils to which the sinuses are connected. The sinus in the cheek bone is known as maxillary sinus, that above the eyes as frontal sinus and the deep one behind the nose as ethmoidal sinus.

There are two forms of sinusitis-Acute and Chronic.

Acute Sinusitis

It is due to an attack of acute rhinitis or, it may occur during the course of influenza. The symptoms are nasal discharge and obstruction. In maxillary sinusitis, the pain may be felt in cheeks, whereas in frontal sinusitis, severe frontal headache is felt. With ethmoiditis, there is pain behind the eyes. Sometimes orbital cellulitis causes severe complications. With sphenoidal sinusitis the characteristic headache is occipital or vertical.

Chronic Sinusitis

It may occur in any or all of the accessory nasal sinuses. It is usually due to an extension of the infection from the nasal cavities. Acute rhinitis or cold in the head is the most frequent cause. Acute specific fevers, injury or operation on the nose are other causes of chronic sinus. Infection of the maxillary sinus frequently follows dental diseases or the extraction of teeth.

The most constant and important symptom is the purulent or mucopurulent discharge from one nostril, which is offensive or sticky. Sometimes discharge is not seen and nasal obstruction is the main complication.

Chronic Maxillary Sinusitis

It's the most common form of sinusitis. The patient complains of discharge in the affected side of the nose & nasal obstruction. Examination shows pus lying under the middle terminate bone. An X-ray picture will show opacity. In ethmoidal and frontal sinusitis, the flow is more in upright position. It comes from under the middle turbinate and there is often pain in the brow and orbit.

Discharge from the posterior ethmoidal and sphenoidal sinuses flows over the middle turbinate and down into the pharynx. Headache is common at the back or top of the head. Various constitutional symptoms due to septic absorption are associated with sinus diseases. Lassitude, headache, occasional elevation of temperature and numerous nervous and vasomotor symptoms are observed. They have a periodic or paroxysmal character. Facial neuralgia may result from sinus diseases. If neglected it may excite middle ear catarrh (with tinitus, deafness etc.), recurrent nasal catarrh and nasal polypi.

General Treatment

In acute attack, inhalation of menthol or tincture benzine is helpful. In maxillary sinusitis sometimes puncture helps favouring drainage from the affected sinus. Sometimes operation for establishing drainage is performed. Deviated septum is seen in chronic form of sinusitis. Ephedrine spray is used and various electrical methods are carried out.

Aconite

Best suited for sudden cold with congestion of the nose, dry, suffocative cold, nose stopped up, scanty watery coryza, sinusitis due to influenza, patient suffering from dry, cold weather, from checked perspiration and also complaints from very hot weather. There is mental and physical restlessness, anguish of mind and a state of fear. Sinusitis with sudden fear.

Arsenic iodide:

Suits well to those who suffer from hay fever, hronic nasal catarrh, swollen nose, thin, watery, ritating, excoriating discharge. Aggravation by neezing.

Ammonium carb

Mucous membranes of the respiratory organs are especially affected. Discharge of sharp burning, water, nose bleed. Nose is stuffy at night with long continued coryza, ozena.

Hepar sulph

The patient is highly susceptible to cold, cannot tolerate fan or air even from the next room. The nose is sore, ulcerative running of the nose. First the discharge is semi liquid, then thick and offensive, tonsillitis, septic sore throat, hay fever etc.

Lemna minor

Suits well when polypi and swollen turbinates are seen. It is useful in atrophic rhinitis. Asthma from nasal obstruction. Dryness of the nasopharynx.

Natrum mur:

Violent, fluent coryza lastinsg from one to three days. Excessive sneezing coryza. Loss of smell and taste due to coryza. Discharge from the nose is watery like raw white of egg. Sinus headache, especially right sided.

Sabadilla:

Spasmodic sneezing with running nose. Copious watery discharge, drops oozing from the tip of the nose, sneezing, running of the eyes with redness.

ULCERATION OF THE NOSE

Is due to syphilitic infection in the early stage of the disease. It causes obstruction in the nose. When children suffer from this trouble congenitally, it is called "Snuffles." The discharge is offensive. Positive Wasserman's reaction helps to fix the diagnosis. In atrophic rhinitis, the odour is foul but there are no ulcers formed in the nose.. The nasal mucous membrane is pale and there is no history of syphilis or tuberculosis in the patient's illness.

Treatment

Arsenic iodide

Thin irritating discharge from anterior and posterior nares, sneezing, hay fever, chronic nasal catarrh, swollen nose, profuse thick yellow discharge. Ulcers, nose excoriated. Sneezing aggravates. Potency 6, 200, 1000.

Kali iodide

Profuse, acrid, watery, coryza, nose red, swollen, tip of nose red, ozena with perforated septum, nasal cold involving frontal sinus. Stiffness and dryness of nose without discharge. Profuse, cool, greenish excoriating discharge It cures syphilitic ulcerations. Potency 6 or 200 and 1000.

Nitric acid

Ozena with green casts in the morning. Coryza with sore & bleeding nostrils, caries of the septum, chronic nasal catarrh with yellow offensive discharge call for this remedy. It is the best remedy in nasal, diphtheria with watery and excoriating discharge. Potency 30, 200.

CONGESTION

The condition of stuffed up nose & inability to breathe freely through the nose arises from many causes. The prominent causes are swollen mucous membrane of the nose, nasal polypi, over grown adenoid glands, deviated septum, sinus trouble and frequent affection of cold. For congestion of nose, we have to select the medicine according to cause. The medicines are already given for above conditions under different chapters according to the disease. The prominent medicines are as follows.

Ammonium carb., Lemna minor, Arum triphyllum, Aconite nap., Belladonna, Ferrum phos., Sambucus, Spongia, Hepar sulph etc.

ANOSMIA

Loss of sense of smell (anosmia) may result from any of the conditions that cause a stuffed up nose. Brain damage or head injuries affecting the olfactory nerve can also be responsible. Drugs like phenol applied to the nose can eliminate the sense of smell. The nerve endings of the olfactory nerve are quickly fatigued. Hence some powerful odours may paralyse the sense of smell. Medicines for loss of smell are:-

Ammonium mur, Alumina, Anacardium, Hepar sulph, Kali bichro, Pulsatilla, Zincum mur, Sanguinaria. The medicine, from the above list may be selected according to the characteristics and general symptoms.

■

THROAT DISEASES

ADENOIDS

These are the glands in clusters of lymph tissue, high in the back of the throat where the nasal passages enter into. The overgrowth of these glands is commonly seen in children. The child breathes with the mouth open and thus acquires a characteristic vacancy of expression. The intellect is often below average. The voice is nasal or dull in character. Snoring and disturbed sleep are the other symptoms. Adenoids may lead to middle ear catarrh and subsequent deafness. Adenoids in the naso-pharynx are usually accompanied by chronic enlargement of the tonsils. The disease often runs in families. Adenoids is supposed to be a form of chronic pharyngitis limited to the naso-pharynx but the lymphoid granulations are seen in the oro-pharynx also. In some children, the shape of the chest becomes narrow and it is called "pigeon chest".

Treatment

Baryta carb

Is very useful in children having a stunted growth due to adenoids and enlarged tonsils. The child is inactive and mentally dull. There is offensive perspiration. It is very useful in suppurative tonsillitis and in infantilism when the memory is weak and the child seems inattentive, stupid and does not learn to play or walk. It is also useful in cretinism and simple goitre.

Agraphis nutans

Best suited to children who suffer from adenoids and enlarged tonsils. Adenoids with deafness. Coryza when the discharge is free. Patient is susceptible to cold.

Calcarea iodatum

Is useful in adenoids & scrofulous affections especially enlarged glands and tonsils. Thyroid enlargement. Flabby children subject to colds. Potency 6, 30 or 200.

Other medicines

Cistus can, Tuberculinum, Calcarea fluor, Calc. phos and Sanguinaria nitrate.

TONSILLITIS

Inflammation of the tonsils is known as 'Tonsillitis'. It may be acute or chronic in nature. Unhygienic conditions such as bad ventilation and overcrowding, bacterial infection from strepto and staphylococcus or pneumococcus cause tonsillitis. Influenza, common cold, rheumatic fever, sore throat, droplet infection especially in schools and public places are the other causes of tonsillitis.

In chronic tonsillitis, running of the nose, fetid breathe, enlarged cervical glands, discharge from the ears and the history of frequent cold will be noticed. Children suffering from chronic tonsillitis are punny and suffer from nervous, respiratory or alimentary disorders.

Treatment

Belladonna

Suits well in acute tonsillitis when the head is hot and the carotids are throbbing. There is great congestion in the throat with angry looking red area. Difficulty in swallowing. Patient is worse while drinking liquids and feels contracted. Scraping sensation and a sensation of a lump in the throat is present.

Apis

Works well when the tonsils are swollen and the surrounding area is puffy. There are ulcers on tonsils, uvula is swollen with stinging pain and construction. The throat is fiery red.

Hepar sulph

Suits well to scrofulous and lymphatic constitutions who are inclined to have glandular swellings and frequent cold. It is a prominent medicine in quinsy i.e. when the tonsils are about to form pus. There is splinter-like sensation in the throat (Nitric acid).

Other medicines

Ferrum phos, Nitric acid, Baryta carb, Sulphur, Phytolacca, Silica and Mercurius vivus.

QUINSY

The condition quinsy or peritonsillar abscess occurs after tonsillitis or sometimes an abscess forms just outside the capsule of the tonsil, usually on one side. Severe pain is felt in the throat and swallowing becomes almost impossible. The pain radiates to the ear and down the neck. The temperature may be high (103° or 104° F) - The patient looks toxic and his speech becomes thick. Trismus (lock jaw) makes the examination difficult. The cervical glands become tender and enlarged.

Medicines

Apis, Hepar sulph, Mercury v, Baryta iod, Silicea.

Baryta iodide works well in 6 potency or if needed in 1000 potency also. Other medicines should, be selected from 30 or 200 potency. Treatment for quinsy and chronic tonsillitis is almost the same.

SORE THROAT

Is a symptom common to nearly all diseases of the throat. The common causes of acute sore throat are:- Common cold, Pharyngitis-both acute and chronic forms, Tonsillitis, Scarlet fever, Diphtheria, Syphilis etc. Rare causes are:- Retro-pharyngeal abscess, Oedema of the throat (acute), Cancer, T. B., and some specific fevers. Chronic sore throat is due to chronic congestion of the organs involved and consequent predisposition to the repeated occurrence of subacute attacks. It forms one variety of Teacher's or Singer's sore throat.

Treatment

Aconite

Suits well in acute sore throat with violent tension in the throat. Complaint caused by exposure to dry, cold weather or draught of cold air, or from very hot weather. It cures influenzal sore throat. Red, burning, dry throat. Potency 200.

Belladonna

Throat is dry as if glazed, angry looking, congestion. Tonsils enlarged with painful deglutition. Hypertrophied mucous membrane of the throat. Potency 30 and 200.

Arum triph

Swelling of sub-maxillary glands, mouth sore and cracked. Hoarseness (loss of voice), teacher's or Clergyman's sore throat. Voice uncertain and worse by talking, singing etc. Useful in catarrhal sore throat. Potency 6 or 200.

Kali bichromicum

Is useful in chronic sore throat. The fauces are red and inflamed, uvula relaxed. Diphtheritic sore throat,

Discharge from mouth and throat is tough and stringy. Voice is hoarse. Potency 6 or 30.

Other Medicines

Hepar sulph, Hydrastis, Ferrum phos, Kali mur etc.

RETRO PHARYNGEAL ABSCESS

This abscess occurs in the areolar tissue between the pharynx and spine. It may develop insidiously or suddenly. It is known by the rigidity of the head with difficult swallowing. Alterations of voice and inspiratory stridor. Posterior pharyngeal wall should be inspected. It is due to acute infection of the nose or, throat or surrounding lymphatic glands. Feeble and rachitic children suffer from this type of abscess.

Treatment

Belladonna

In acute attack. Should be given in 200 potency if its usual symptoms are present.

Other Medicines

Hepar sulph, Lachesis, Silica, Mercury, Antipyrin. In surgical cases, anesthesia is not given.

DIPHTHERIA

Diphtheria is an acute infectious disease caused by a specific germ-the diphtheria bacillus. It is characterised by patches of a greenish membrane on the tonsils or throat. If not treated well in time, this membrane can choke the patient to death. The disease is most common in children and prevalent especially in winter season. Every infant at 6 months should be immunized against this dreadful disease.

Symptoms

Sore throat from the beginning. Then there is inability to swallow. But in young children both these symptoms are often absent. A patch of creamy white or grayish colour is seen in one or both tonsils. The patient feels his neck stir, and the glands of the jaw are swollen. Prostration and anaemia are prominent symptoms, but the mind is usually clear. In severe attacks oedema round the neck is observed and it is known as "Bull-Neck." In fatal cases, purpuric rash or erythema on the skin is seen. The disease occurs chiefly in young children especially under 10 years of age. Whooping cough, measles and certain acute infectious are the predisposing causes. The disease spreads by droplet infection from person to person. It is conveyed by infected handkerchiefs, cups, spoons etc. Milk is also a carrier. The main complication of diphtheria is paralysis.

Treatment

Lachesis

Sore throat. Worse left side and swallowing liquids. It cure's septic parotiditis, diphtheria. Membrane dusky blackish. Pain is aggravated by hot drinks. It cannot be forced up or down. Throat is very painful. It is worse on slightest touch or pressure. The trouble starts on the left and then extends to the right. Tonsils are purple. Pains into ear. Collar and neck band must be very loose. It cures diphtheritic paralysis. Potency 30 and 200.

Mercurius bin iodide

Is useful when the sub-maxillary glands are painfully enlarged. Worse on left tonsil, aphonia. Diphtheria and ulcerated sore throat. Potency 3 or 6.

Mercurius cyanatus

This is proved to be a most efficacious medicine in diphtheria. Intense redness of throat; swallowing difficult. Diphtheria of the larynx and nose. Potency 3 or 6.

Echinacea

This medicine is a blood corrector. It cures ulcers of the throat. Gray exudations in the posterior nares and air passages. Gangrene, blood poisoning and septic conditions. Potency 30, 200, 1000.

Apis mel.

The throat is red, shining and puffy. Membrane of the mouth and throat seems glossy. There are stinging pains. The gums and lips are swollen. Oedema in the pharynx. Potency 200

Phytolacca

Sore throat, quinsy, diphtheria. Throat is dark red or bluish red, Soft palate and tonsils are swollen. Throat feels rough, narrow, hot. Pseudo-membranous deposits, greenish, thick, white, tenacious, yellowish mucus, difficult to expectorate. It cures mumps and diphtheria. Potency 6, 30, 200,

PHARYNGITIS

Is an inflammation of mucous membrane of pharynx and soft palate and to a certain extent of the tonsils also. In mild cases, the symptoms are - dryness of the throat, slight discomfort in swallowing, tickling and hawking etc. But in severe cases, there may be oedema and severe congestion in the throat. The disease lasts for few days ending generally in resolution and sometimes passes into a chronic condition.

Chronic Pharyngitis

There are two varieties of chronic pharyngitis. 1) Catarrhal (2) Granular (Follicular). Chronic catarrhal variety presents the same symptoms of the acute type, but in a milder degree and for a prolonged period. It is also known as relapsing sore throat due to chronic congestion, of the throat. It forms one variety of Clergyman's or school teacher's sore throat.

Granular Pharyngitis

Is a chronic condition having granulation on the pharyngeal walls due to the grouping of masses of lymphoid cells around the opening of the ducts of the mucous glands. The ducts may become obstructed and dilated later causing yellow discharge and cheesy material and the condition is named as Follicular pharyngitis.

A patient suffers from repeated attacks of sore throat especially in the morning and leads to chronic cough and hawking. When a disease continues for a long time, that becomes dry from atrophy of the glands (Pharyngitis sicca) Infection in the nose also helps in keeping the condition prolonged.

Treatment

Aconite

Useful in acute pharyngitis with burning in the throat. Tonsils swollen and dry. The mouth is red dry and constricted. Prickling & stinging in the throat. Potency 200.

Bryonia

Tongue coated white, dry cough, pain in the chest on spell of coughing, headache. Patient is worse by motion and better while at rest. Potency 30, 200.

Ferrum phos

Mouth hot, fauces red inflamed, ulcerated, sort throat. Tonsils red and swollen. Eustachian tubes inflamed. Sore throat of singers. Sub-acute laryngitis with red throat (use 2x). After operations of nose and throat to control bleeding and relieve soreness. First stage of inflammation. Potency 3x, 200, 1000.

Kali bichromicum

Is useful in cases of chronic pharyngitis when the throat is congested, red and rough. Parotid glands swollen. Uvula relaxed, oedematous and bladder-like. Pseudo membranous deposits on the tonsils and soft. Palate, Potency 6, 30, 200.

Senega

Is useful in catarrhal pharyngitis with cough especially in old aged patients. It is useful in pharyngitis and laryngitis with hoarseness and cough, Potency 3, 6, 30.

LARYNGITIS

Acute laryngitis is especially seen in children when it is described as 'croup' in which a child wakes up suddenly at night with loud inspiratory sound (stridor) followed by an attack of coughing (laryngitis stridulus)

Causes of acute laryngitis

Exposure to cold combined with over-use and wrong production of the voice (Actors, Singers etc.). It is frequently a part of the 'common cold'. Measles and diphtheria may cause laryngitis. A foreign body in the larynx or 'trachea is cause of irritation resembling laryngitis.

Chronic Laryngitis

Is troublesome on account of perpetual hoarseness and liability to acute attacks.

Causes

(1) Repeated acute attacks, (2) Excessive speaking, teaching, singing, over-use with faulty production of voice. (3) Dusty air, (4) Nasal obstruction and mouth breathing. (5) T. B. Syphilis, ulcerations and new growth. In cases of intractable laryngitis the above causes should be kept in mind. (6) Nasal sinusitis, (7) Spread of inflammation from adjacent areas. (Granular pharyngitis etc). (8) Rheumatic and gouty constitutions do get laryngitis.

Treatment

Aconite

In acute catarrhal laryngitis with fever, voice husky. Can scarcely speak, inhalation difficult and noisy. Use 200.

Apis

Oedema in the larynx with painful suffocative cough and great dyspnoea, laryngitis with erysipelas. Often indicated when Belladonna fails. Potency 30, 200.

Argentum nitricum

Is useful in chronic laryngitis of singers. Raising the voice causes cough, hoarseness and loss of voice. Pain and soreness in the throat. There is much hawking. Potency 3, 6. 200,

Allium cepa

Violent catarrhal laryngitis, hoarse cough, watering of the eye, oppressed in the chest. Potency 3, 6, 200.

Kali iodatum

Is efficacious in follicular laryngitis. Laryngitis due to syphilis with deposits in the throat. Green sputa like soap suds, laryngeal phthisis, odema of larynx. Potency 6, 200, 1000.

Lachesis

Is useful in malignant type of laryngitis. Oedema, very sensitive to touch, nasal speech, suffocation. Potency 30, 200.

Spongia

Goitre, laryngitis, phthisis, whistling and rattling from the larynx. Potency 6, 30, 200.

Other Medicines

Belladonna, Causticum, Ammonium carb, Drosera, Hepar sulph, Kali bi. Mercurius, Rumex and Phosphorus.

Some Clinical Experiences

In cases of discharges from the ears, I have found the following, medicines very useful.

Hepar sulph 200

When the discharge is partly watery and partly purulent. In such patients, the cause of the ailment would be exposure to cold, enlarged septic tonsils, fevers and the patient's great susceptibility to cold - a characteristic of Hepar sulph constitution. Calcarea sulph is found very useful when the discharge is mixed with blood. There is tendency to form blood boils in the ear and it goes on suppurating pending the recovery for a prolonged time. In such cases, I have found Calc. sulph a wonder drug, I use 6, 30 or 200 potency. In chronic cases, 1000 or C. M. (one lakh potency) potencies are found useful. Sometimes I prescribe biochemic medicines such as Ferrum phos, Kali mur and Silica in 3x or 30x potencies.

I have treated a case of chronic mastoiditis with otosclerosis. She was a lady 42 years old coming from Bombay. She was treated by leading E. N. T. specialists from Bombay and other places in Maharashtra. Her X-rays were taken and the findings clearly showed the bony tissue changes that had occured in the internal ear. She was worried as nobody could cure her ailment — especially the offensive discharge from her ears. She came to me with the hope of last efforts. I was treating her for a long time and could cure her completely after giving trials to different homoeopathic medicines. The medicines given from time to time were Capsicum, Calc. sulph, Calc. fluor, Silicea, Asafoetida, Pulsatilla etc.

A Case of Tinitus

I have cured a case of tinitus of a patient aged about 64. He had aural vertigo and hissing sounds in the ears causing sleeplessness. He was cured by giving Chininum sulph 6 potency.

A Case of Chronic pharyngitis and Laryngitis.

It was a very interesting case of a lady. She was a princess and ultimately a sort of a "customer" to many leading doctors. She was given different antibiotics. Some suggested different operations of nose, tonsils and throat. Some doctors left it as incurable. Finally she got my address and narrated me the history of her case. I told her frankly that there is no need of any operation and that she should have great patience to undergo the homoeopathic treatment as her case was mal-treated and quite chronic also. She agreed to my words and took the medicines faithfully and totally got cured after a prolonged treatment. The medicines given in her case were Kali bichromicum, Hydrastis, Nitric acid, Sulphur. Kreosote, Arum triph, Thuja, Am. carb; Nux vomica etc. Her trouble of leucorrhea and vaginitis was also treated at the same time and the results were good.

A Case of Ozena - A Male Patient Aged 34. He was getting chronic offensive discharge from nose and formation of scabs. He was highly perturbed as the disease was not only troublesome to him but to others also due to foul nasal discharge. He was cured by following medicines Kali iodatum 6. Hippozaenia 30. (cured the case 90%) Cadmium sulph, Hepar sulph 200 and Aurum met 6 & 200 potency.

+++